USING

N-ACETYL CYSTEINE

FOR BEGINNERS

Essential Primer To Boost Your Health Vitality, Liver Support Wellness, Well-Being And More

DR. SPARKS RUBIO

Copyright © Sparks Rubio, 2023

All rights reserved. No part of this book may be reproduced or transmitted in any form or by any means, electronic or mechanical, including photocopying, recording, or by any information storage and retrieval system, without permission in writing from the author, except for brief quotations embodied in critical reviews and certain other noncommercial uses permitted by copyright law.

DISCLAIMER

The information presented in this book is intended for general informational purposes only. It is not a substitute for professional medical advice, diagnosis, or treatment.

The author and publisher of this book have made every effort to ensure that the information provided is accurate and up-to-date at the time of publication. However, medical and scientific knowledge is constantly evolving, and new research may emerge. Therefore, the information in this book should not be considered a definitive source for medical or nutritional advice.

It is essential to consult with a qualified healthcare professional before making any decisions.

The author and publisher disclaim any liability for any adverse outcomes or consequences resulting from the use or misuse of the information in this book. Readers are urged to use their discretion and judgment when making decisions about their health and wellness.

By reading this book, you agree to do so at your own risk and should not use it as a substitute for professional medical advice or treatment.

TABLE OF CONTENTS

- INTRODUCTION TO N-ACETYL CYSTEINE (NAC) 8
  - ACKNOWLEDGMENTS 8
  - SUPPLEMENTS' PLACE IN TODAY'S HEALTH 10
  - DEFINITION OF N-ACETYL CYSTEINE (NAC) 12
  - GOALS FOR THIS BOOK 14
- CHAPTER ONE 16
  - KNOWLEDGE OF N-ACETYL CYSTEINE 16
    - HISTORY AND ORIGIN 16
    - CYSTEINE VERSUS NAC 17
    - NAC AS A GLUTATHIONE PRECURSOR: 18
    - PRINCIPLES OF ACTION: 19
- CHAPTER TWO 22
  - NAC'S HEALTH BENEFITS 22
    - OXIDANT CHARACTERISTICS 22
    - DETOXING AND SUPPORT FOR THE LIVER 23
    - BREATHING HEALTH 24
    - NEUROPSYCHIATRY AND NAC 25
    - ADDITIONAL POTENTIAL HEALTH 27
- CHAPTER THREE 28
  - NAC AND HEALTH ISSUES 28

- NAC IN CYSTIC FIBROSIS 28
- CHRONIC OBSTRUCTIVE PULMONARY DISEASE AND NAC 29
- NAC IN OVERDOSAGE OF ACETAMINOPHEN 31
- NAC AND DISORDERS OF THE MIND 32

CHAPTER FOUR 34
- USING NAC IN FOOD SUPPLEMENTS 34
  - TYPES OF SUPPLEMENTAL NAC..............................34
  - RECOMMENDED DOSAGE......................................35
  - POSSIBLE ADVERSE REACTIONS AND SAFETY 36
  - INTERACTIONS BETWEEN DRUGS 37
  - ASPECTS OF PURCHASING AND QUALITY TO 38

CHAPTER FIVE 40
- INVESTIGATIONS AND SCHOLARLY RESEARCH 40
  - A SYNOPSIS OF NAC STUDIES................................40
  - POSITIVE CLINICAL TRIAL RESULTS........................41
  - CURRENT RESEARCH AND UPCOMING 42
  - LIMITATIONS AND DISPUTES 44

CHAPTER SIX 46
- INCLUDING NAC IN YOUR DAILY WELLNESS PRACTICE 46

- SPEAKING WITH A MEDICAL PROFESSIONAL 46
- TAILORED APPLICATION AND ADVANTAGES 47
- BLENDING NAC WITH ADDITIONAL 49
- LIFESTYLE POINTS TO CONSIDER: 51
- CHAPTER SEVEN 54
  - THE MODERN WORLD OF NAC 54
    - NAC IN EXERCISE AND SPORTS 54
    - ENVIRONMENTAL AND ETHICAL 55
    - NAC IN RECIPES & COOKING 57
    - MAKE YOUR BEAUTY PRODUCTS 58
    - PROBLEMS 60
    - POLICY AND REGULATORY CONSIDERATIONS 61

INTRODUCTION TO N-ACETYL CYSTEINE (NAC)

ACKNOWLEDGMENTS

The process of writing a thorough book is never an isolated undertaking; rather, it is the result of the help and direction provided by many people and organizations. I sincerely thank everyone who helped make this project a reality. I am truly grateful for their contributions. First and foremost, I would like to express my gratitude to my family, whose continuous support and faith in my goals have been the foundation of my quest for knowledge. Their tolerance and comprehension have been essential in giving me the time and room to explore the intricacies of this topic.

In addition, I would want to convey my sincere gratitude to my mentors and advisors, whose insight and counsel have molded my comprehension and viewpoint. Their astute comments and helpful critiques have been immensely helpful in honing the theories and concepts covered in this book. I owe a debt of gratitude as well to the academics, specialists, and researchers whose groundbreaking work made it possible to explore the themes covered in these pages.

SUPPLEMENTS' PLACE IN TODAY'S HEALTH

The role of supplements has drawn a lot of interest and attention in light of the rapidly changing modern healthcare landscape. Supplements have emerged as a key component in the quest for optimum health and well-being, containing a diverse range of vitamins, minerals, herbs, and other substances. Dietary supplements are becoming a well-liked option for people looking to fill in nutritional deficiencies and support different physiological functions as the emphasis on preventative healthcare grows. Furthermore, the investigation of supplements as a supplement to traditional medical procedures has been accelerated by the growing interest in holistic well-being and the integration of complementary medicine.

Notably, supplements are becoming more widely acknowledged for their ability to support certain body functions and mitigate deficits, which can help maintain general health. They work as a supplemental strategy to support physiological processes that may be hampered by a variety of variables, including food, lifestyle, and environmental impacts, and to alleviate nutritional deficiencies. A thorough understanding of supplements' mechanisms of action, efficacy, and potential interactions in the context of modern healthcare practices is imperative, given their pivotal role in promoting health and wellness.

DEFINITION OF N-ACETYL CYSTEINE (NAC)

Natural amino acid derivative N-acetyl cysteine (NAC) is a strong antioxidant with a wide range of medicinal uses that have attracted a lot of interest. Noted for its capacity to restore intracellular glutathione levels, NAC is an important precursor for the manufacture of this molecule, which is necessary for the preservation of cellular integrity and redox balance. Due to its complex pharmacological characteristics, it has been the focus of much research in several disciplines, including neurology, psychiatry, and pulmonology.

Apart from its function as an antecedent of glutathione, NAC demonstrates an array of biological actions that culminate in its capacity as a mucolytic agent. This ability to facilitate mucus production is particularly useful in the treatment of respiratory disorders. Furthermore, studies into its therapeutic potential in treating psychiatric illnesses like addiction, bipolar disorder, and obsessive-compulsive disorder (OCD) have been inspired by its capacity to modulate neurotransmitter levels. The wide range of biological effects exhibited by NAC highlights its potential as a therapeutic agent, hence necessitating a thorough investigation of its mechanisms of action and clinical utility in the context of contemporary healthcare.

GOALS FOR THIS BOOK

The goals of this book are to clarify the complex world of supplements, specifically N-Acetyl Cysteine (NAC), within the framework of modern health and wellness regimens. This book aims to provide a thorough understanding of the function of supplements in boosting general health while shining light on the complex mechanisms underlying the therapeutic potential of NAC by combining scientific insights, clinical evidence, and practical applications. By investigating its pharmacological characteristics, therapeutic uses, and possible drawbacks, this book seeks to provide a comprehensive overview of the use of NAC as an adjunctive strategy to address a range of health issues.

CHAPTER ONE

KNOWLEDGE OF N-ACETYL CYSTEINE

HISTORY AND ORIGIN

The use of N-acetyl cysteine (NAC) as a mucolytic drug to treat respiratory disorders began in the 1960s, and its history is extensive. It was initially used mainly to treat people with chronic bronchitis and other lung conditions to thin and loosen their mucus. Researchers eventually started to learn more about its complex qualities and its therapeutic uses in addition to its original purpose. Because of its adaptability, it has been investigated in psychiatry, neurology, and general medicine, among other medical specialties.

CYSTEINE VERSUS NAC

The amino acid L-cysteine is changed to become NAC, which is different from its precursor in numerous important ways. When compared to L-cysteine alone, the cysteine molecule has an acetyl group connected to it, which increases its stability and bioavailability and increases its effectiveness when taken orally. While the functions of both substances as antioxidants and protein building blocks are identical,

NAC has clear benefits in terms of cell transport and absorption, making it more useful as a medication in some situations.

NAC AS A GLUTATHIONE PRECURSOR:

The fact that NAC functions as a precursor to glutathione, an essential antioxidant produced by the body, is one of its most noteworthy qualities. Glutathione is essential for the defense of cells against oxidative stress, which is linked to several disease processes. NAC acts as a direct precursor, which helps to restore intracellular glutathione. This function is especially important in diseases of the liver, brain problems, and some respiratory ailments where oxidative damage plays a major role. Because NAC raises glutathione levels, it is being investigated as a possible medicinal drug to treat a variety of illnesses.

PRINCIPLES OF ACTION:

NAC has a wide range of therapeutic applications since it works through many processes. Donating sulfhydryl groups allows it to function as a precursor for the manufacture of glutathione, which is one of the main mechanisms. NAC promotes cellular detoxification mechanisms and reduces oxidative stress by raising glutathione levels. Furthermore, it has been discovered that NAC alters the action of several neurotransmitters, such as glutamate, which may have consequences for its application in neurological and psychiatric conditions. Furthermore, NAC exhibits anti-inflammatory qualities, which are explained by its capacity to suppress reactive oxygen species and pro-inflammatory cytokines.

CHAPTER TWO
NAC'S HEALTH BENEFITS
OXIDANT CHARACTERISTICS

The well-known vitamin N-acetylcysteine (NAC) is well-known for its many health advantages. One of its main characteristics is that it's a noteworthy antioxidant. NAC mitigates oxidative stress and aids in the neutralization of free radicals since it is a precursor to glutathione, an extremely potent antioxidant. This procedure aids in cell damage prevention, which may reduce the chance of chronic illnesses linked to oxidative stress, including cancer, heart disease, and neurological disorders. Moreover, people whose antioxidant defenses have been weakened by a variety of medical illnesses or lifestyle choices may benefit especially from NAC's capacity to restore glutathione levels.

DETOXING AND SUPPORT FOR THE LIVER

The detoxifying and liver-supporting qualities of NAC have drawn interest from medical professionals. By increasing the synthesis of glutathione, a crucial element in the liver's detoxification process, it helps break down certain poisons. NAC may lessen the load on the liver and assist its optimal operation by encouraging the removal of toxic chemicals. This characteristic is particularly important because of the liver's primary function in the metabolism of several substances, drugs, and environmental pollutants that can build up in the body over time.

BREATHING HEALTH

In terms of respiratory health, NAC has demonstrated potential in the treatment of bronchitis, cystic fibrosis, and chronic obstructive pulmonary disease (COPD). Because of its mucolytic qualities, mucus is easier to thin and release from the respiratory tract. Furthermore, because of its antioxidant qualities, the lungs experience less inflammation and oxidative damage, which may help manage respiratory symptoms and enhance lung function overall. Though more research is required to determine its effectiveness in various respiratory disorders, the evidence that is currently available points to a beneficial effect.

NEUROPSYCHIATRY AND NAC

Regarding mental health, NAC has garnered interest because of its plausible involvement in a range of neurological and psychiatric conditions. Research has indicated that it may help treat symptoms related to disorders like schizophrenia, bipolar disorder, and obsessive-compulsive disorder (OCD). It is thought that NAC's ability to modulate dopaminergic and glutamatergic pathways contributes to its therapeutic promise in treating specific cognitive and behavioral disorders. Additionally, because of its antioxidant qualities, it might be able to lessen the oxidative stress that is linked to the pathophysiology of several mental health conditions.

ADDITIONAL POTENTIAL HEALTH ADVANTAGES

NAC has demonstrated potential in several additional health domains in addition to its well-established roles. According to some research, it may help maintain cardiovascular health by assisting in blood pressure and cholesterol balance. Studies exploring its possible use in the treatment of inflammatory diseases like arthritis have also been prompted by its anti-inflammatory qualities.

CHAPTER THREE
NAC AND HEALTH ISSUES
NAC IN CYSTIC FIBROSIS

N-acetylcysteine, or NAC, has shown therapeutic promise in several medical problems. Because of its diverse pharmacological characteristics, it is a prospective drug for several illnesses. NAC's mucolytic and antioxidant qualities have drawn interest in the setting of cystic fibrosis (CF). A genetic illness called cystic fibrosis (CF) is characterized by unusually thick and sticky mucus production, which can cause serious respiratory difficulties.

The mucolytic activity of NAC helps to lower mucus viscosity, which makes it easier for the mucus to be cleared from the airways. Furthermore, because of its antioxidant properties, CF patients may have improved lung function and a slower rate of disease progression by reducing the oxidative stress that is frequently linked to the disease.

CHRONIC OBSTRUCTIVE PULMONARY DISEASE AND NAC

Research on the therapeutic effects of NAC has been focused on Chronic Obstructive Pulmonary Disease (COPD), a progressive respiratory illness characterized by inflammation, oxidative stress, and airflow limitation. Because of its mucolytic qualities, NAC helps improve expectoration and reduce the viscosity of sputum, which improves lung function and may lessen the frequency and intensity of exacerbations in COPD patients. Additionally, it is thought that its ant oxidative properties help to lessen oxidative damage and inflammation in the lungs, which may enhance the quality of life for COPD patients generally.

NAC IN OVERDOSAGE OF ACETAMINOPHEN

NAC is an essential counteragent for acetaminophen (paracetamol) overdose. Overdosing on acetaminophen can cause damage to the liver; early NAC delivery has been demonstrated to prevent or reduce the severity of hepatotoxicity. In the end, NAC protects the liver from the harmful consequences of the overdose by acting as a precursor for glutathione, an essential antioxidant in the liver that is needed to restore glutathione levels and improve the detoxification of the poisonous metabolite of acetaminophen.

NAC AND DISORDERS OF THE MIND

There is also a lot of curiosity about how NAC might be used to treat specific mental health disorders. Research indicates that NAC could have positive benefits on diseases such as substance use disorders, schizophrenia, bipolar disorder, and obsessive-compulsive disorder (OCD). Some patients may experience improved symptoms and cognitive function as a result of its putative neuroprotective and neuromodulatory effects, which are thought to be influenced by its modulation of glutamatergic, dopaminergic, and neuroinflammatory pathways.

Although further investigation is required to determine its exact modes of action and effectiveness in various mental health disorders, existing data suggests that it may have a promising future as an adjuvant treatment option.

CHAPTER FOUR

USING NAC IN FOOD SUPPLEMENTS

TYPES OF SUPPLEMENTAL NAC

A dietary supplement called N-acetylcysteine (NAC) has attracted a lot of interest due to its possible health advantages. It is a modified version of the amino acid cysteine, which is essential for several body processes, most notably the synthesis of the potent antioxidant glutathione. As a nutritional supplement, NAC comes in several forms, such as liquid formulations, powders, pills, and capsules. These forms provide users with the freedom to select the most practical mode of absorption based on personal preferences and particular health concerns.

RECOMMENDED DOSAGE

When it comes to dose recommendations, the right amount of NAC to take as a dietary supplement depends on several variables, such as the goal of the supplementing, specific medical problems, and medical professional guidance. Although a set standard dosage has not been defined, normal doses are divided into many administrations and range from 600 to 1800 milligrams per day. It is essential to follow the suggested dosage recommendations and speak with a healthcare provider, particularly when thinking about larger dosages or longer use.

POSSIBLE ADVERSE REACTIONS AND SAFETY MEASURES

When used in the recommended dosages, NAC is generally thought to be safe for the majority of individuals; however, it's vital to be aware of potential adverse effects and take precautions. Some people could get mild gastrointestinal symptoms such as diarrhea, vomiting, or nausea. Furthermore, uncommon allergic responses or breathing problems in susceptible people have been documented. Before taking NAC, people who have a history of asthma or peptic ulcers should use caution and speak with a healthcare professional because NAC may make these illnesses worse.

INTERACTIONS BETWEEN DRUGS

Because NAC supplementation may decrease the effectiveness of medications that contain nitroglycerin, activated charcoal, or both, those using these substances should avoid it due to potential medication interactions. Furthermore, it should be noted that NAC may interfere with some chemotherapy treatments and pharmaceuticals that are processed by the liver. For these reasons, seeking medical advice is essential before adding NAC to a regular supplement regimen.

ASPECTS OF PURCHASING AND QUALITY TO CONSIDER

Prioritizing quality and safety is crucial when thinking about buying NAC supplements. Choosing reliable brands that follow good manufacturing principles (GMP) and go through independent testing to ensure purity and potency will help lower the likelihood of consuming inferior goods. To further guarantee the product's legitimacy and quality, look for any potential allergies or additions in the ingredient list and see if it has a third-party certification seal. Customers should also be on the lookout for fake goods and only buy NAC supplements from reliable sources, such as accredited internet sellers, health stores, and certified pharmacies with a track record of offering real dietary supplements.

CHAPTER FIVE

INVESTIGATIONS AND SCHOLARLY RESEARCH

A SYNOPSIS OF NAC STUDIES

N-acetylcysteine (NAC) research has attracted a lot of interest because of its many potential applications in treating a range of illnesses. NAC's initial focus was on treating acetaminophen toxicity, but it has since broadened to include a variety of possible therapeutic uses. The effects of NAC on oxidative stress, neurotransmission, and immune system regulation have been well-researched. NAC is a major source of glutathione, an antioxidant, and an amino acid precursor. Notably, studies examining its effectiveness in a variety of illnesses, from respiratory ailments to psychiatric problems, have been prompted by its various methods of action.

POSITIVE CLINICAL TRIAL RESULTS

Positive clinical trials have highlighted NAC's potential for treating a variety of illnesses. Studies in the field of psychiatric health have demonstrated its ability to lessen symptoms associated with conditions like obsessive-compulsive disorder, schizophrenia, and bipolar disorder. Because of its capacity to reduce neuroinflammation and oxidative stress, NAC can potentially treat neurodegenerative illnesses by modulating the glutamatergic and dopaminergic systems. Additionally, although more research is needed, its application as an adjuvant therapy in the treatment of addictive behaviors and substance dependence has shown encouraging outcomes.

CURRENT RESEARCH AND UPCOMING PROJECTS

The investigation of NAC's ability to lessen the negative effects of heavy metals and environmental pollutants is gaining momentum in light of current studies and prospective future possibilities. Furthermore, research is being done aggressively to determine how it affects diabetes and metabolic syndrome, as well as how it helps to mitigate insulin resistance. Furthermore, because NAC is an immunological modulator and can affect cellular redox balance and inflammatory pathways, there is interest in using it to treat chronic inflammatory diseases and autoimmune illnesses. Additionally, research is being conducted to explore the possibility of NAC as an adjuvant medicine for cancer treatment, with a focus on improving the effectiveness of chemotherapy and lowering its side effects.

LIMITATIONS AND DISPUTES

NAC study is not without its limitations and disagreements, though. Further standardized clinical studies are necessary since, despite their encouraging results, inconsistent research design, doses, and treatment durations have produced variable outcomes. Furthermore, questions have been raised about the long-term safety of NAC supplementation, especially when high doses are involved, emphasizing the importance of carefully assessing any negative effects. In addition, NAC's unpredictable absorption and possible drug interactions make careful use of the supplement in clinical settings necessary. Furthermore, there are ongoing discussions on the use of NAC as a preventive measure. Given its prophylactic significance in several illnesses, more substantial evidence is required before firm recommendations can be made. To fully utilize NAC's therapeutic potential, it is imperative to overcome the disputes and restrictions that arise when researchers delve deeper into the compound's complex mechanisms and applications.

CHAPTER SIX

INCLUDING NAC IN YOUR DAILY WELLNESS PRACTICE

SPEAKING WITH A MEDICAL PROFESSIONAL

You must have a comprehensive conversation with a licensed healthcare provider before adding NAC (N-Acetyl Cysteine) to your wellness regimen. This consultation is essential because it can provide you with information about your particular health condition, possible drug interactions, and the right dosage based on your unique requirements. Since various people may respond differently to NAC, particularly those who already have health issues, speaking with a healthcare provider can guarantee a safe and customized method of incorporating NAC into your wellness routine. In addition, medical experts can provide direction about the length of use and possible hazards related to its intake, thus promoting an informed decision-making process.

TAILORED APPLICATION AND ADVANTAGES

Optimizing the benefits of NAC requires customizing its utilization to each individual's needs. NAC is well-known for its antioxidant qualities and for helping the body produce glutathione, an essential antioxidant that is involved in many physiological functions. This may be especially helpful for people whose detoxification systems are impaired or who have been exposed to pollutants in the environment. Moreover, NAC has been connected to respiratory health, demonstrating potential in treating ailments such as chronic bronchitis and bolstering respiratory function in those with certain lung-related problems. Furthermore, a preliminary study indicates that it may have the ability to enhance mental health by regulating neurotransmitter levels, which may assist those who are dealing with specific mood-related issues. A more focused and successful health approach may result from knowing the precise advantages that a person is looking for from NAC and adjusting one's use of it accordingly.

BLENDING NAC WITH ADDITIONAL SUPPLEMENTS

Including NAC in your wellness regimen may require you to take into account the supplements' synergistic effects while taking them together. Alpha-lipoic acid and selenium are two substances that stimulate glutathione synthesis; when combined, they may enhance the antioxidant qualities and general health advantages of NAC due to their role in increasing glutathione production. Furthermore, some research indicates that taking NAC along with specific vitamins, including C and E, may improve its antioxidant properties and promote its function in preserving cellular health. Combination therapy should be used carefully though, as some supplements may interact with NAC and change its bioavailability or cause unanticipated negative effects. To optimize NAC's beneficial effects on a person's wellness regimen, it can be difficult to combine it with other supplements. Seeking advice from a trained nutritionist or healthcare provider can assist.

LIFESTYLE POINTS TO CONSIDER:

A comprehensive approach that includes lifestyle adjustments should be incorporated into the integration of NAC into a comprehensive wellness routine. Stressing the importance of a healthy, well-balanced diet full of fruits, vegetables, and whole grains might enhance the benefits of NAC by promoting a strong antioxidant defense system. The benefits of NAC on numerous physiological processes can be enhanced and the body's general resilience reinforced by frequent exercise and upholding a healthy body weight. Furthermore, embracing stress-reduction practices like yoga or mindfulness meditation can support the holistic wellness objectives made possible by NAC in a complementary way, particularly when it comes to the possible advantages for mental health. Moreover, limiting exposure to dangerous chemicals and environmental contaminants might enhance the protective benefits of NAC on the body's detoxifying processes. Including these lifestyle factors can enhance the effectiveness of NAC as a cornerstone of a well-rounded wellness regimen.

CHAPTER SEVEN

THE MODERN WORLD OF NAC

NAC IN EXERCISE AND SPORTS

Because of its potential advantages for athletes and fitness enthusiasts, N-acetyl Cysteine (NAC) has gained attention in the sports and fitness community. Its capacity to increase the body's synthesis of glutathione, a potent antioxidant, is one of its main qualities. Enhancing the body's defense mechanism, NAC can help lower oxidative stress brought on by exercise—a common occurrence during strenuous workouts? Its ability to reduce muscular fatigue and hasten muscle recovery further makes it an appealing supplement for athletes who follow intense training schedules. Many athletes are becoming more interested in including NAC in their diets and supplement regimens, even though research on the substance's direct effects on sports performance is still underway.

ENVIRONMENTAL AND ETHICAL CONSIDERATIONS

Concerns regarding NAC's ethical manufacture and environmental impact have emerged as demand for the product rises. Natural sources including plant extracts and animal byproducts are the source of NAC.

The sourcing of NAC obtained from animals raises ethical questions, highlighting the importance of ethical and sustainable methods in the animal husbandry sector. Moreover, chemical procedures that can be harmful to the environment may be used in the manufacture of NAC. Raw material procurement that is ethical and the use of environmentally friendly production techniques have grown in importance for both customers and producers. As a result, the NAC industry is prioritizing the adoption of sustainable practices and pushing for supply chain transparency to reduce its environmental impact and guarantee that ethical standards are upheld.

NAC IN RECIPES & COOKING

NAC has been included in a wide range of cooking methods and recipes in the culinary arts because of its adaptable qualities and possible health advantages. Because of its capacity to reduce oxidative stress, NAC is becoming more and more common in health-conscious recipes, particularly those that highlight the use of natural antioxidants. Cooking using NAC-rich items increases the nutritional content of food while also improving its flavor profile, such as onions and garlic. Furthermore, NAC is a viable ingredient for recipes requiring heating or lengthy cooking processes due to its durability under specific cooking circumstances. NAC has shown its versatility and potential in the culinary world as chefs and home cooks have started experimenting with inventive ways to include it in both savory and sweet meals.

MAKE YOUR BEAUTY PRODUCTS

In the field of natural skincare and well-being, adding NAC to handmade beauty products has gained popularity. Thanks to its reputation as an antioxidant, NAC is now a highly sought-after component for DIY face masks, serums, and creams. Because of its ability to prevent oxidative damage and encourage skin renewal, it is now regarded as an important ingredient in formulas for anti-aging and skin-brightening products. NAC may help make nourishing and energizing beauty products that appeal to people looking for chemical-free skincare remedies when paired with other natural components like aloe Vera, honey, or essential oils. The DIY method also permits customization, allowing people to fit beauty items to their skin type and requirements.

PROBLEMS

Notwithstanding its auspicious prospects, integrating NAC into different aspects of contemporary life presents considerable obstacles. The control and uniformity of NAC supplements and goods is one of these issues. Securing the quality, safety, and purity of NAC in various industries continues to be a major challenge, necessitating strict regulatory frameworks and industry-wide compliance requirements. Furthermore, those with limited means may find it difficult to fully utilize the advantages of NAC due to the cost and accessibility of goods based on this component. Moreover, misperceptions or a lack of knowledge about the benefits and appropriate applications of NAC can result in abuse or overconsumption, highlighting the necessity of thorough education and awareness efforts to encourage the responsible and knowledgeable use of NAC in a variety of contexts. It is essential to address these issues if NAC is to be fully utilized while protecting the health and welfare of its users.

POLICY AND REGULATORY CONSIDERATIONS

The regulatory and policy aspects significantly influence the structure that companies and sectors' function in. Ensuring equitable competition and safeguarding consumer rights are fundamental aspects of a secure and moral business environment. Policies and regulations establish the bar for ethical behavior and direct company operations in a variety of fields, including banking, healthcare, technology, and the environment.

The financial sector relies heavily on regulatory supervision to protect the economy's stability. To reduce the impact of prospective market downturns and prevent systemic risks, policies including capital requirements, stress testing, and prohibitions on hazardous financial instruments are in place. Furthermore, regulatory agencies and central banks frequently collaborate closely to develop monetary policies that support economic expansion while reducing inflationary pressures, guaranteeing a balance between stability and growth.

Upholding patient safety, data privacy, and ethical standards in medical practice are the goals of regulatory and policy concerns in the field of healthcare. Before pharmaceuticals and medical equipment are approved for sale, they must pass strict protocols that guarantee their safety and efficacy to the highest levels. Furthermore, privacy laws like the United States' Health Insurance Portability and Accountability Act (HIPAA) safeguard patients' private information while fostering confidence between patients and healthcare providers.

The regulatory environment in the technology sector is nevertheless changing quickly, reflecting the difficulties brought on by new digital breakthroughs. Data protection laws have been implemented to improve individuals' control over their data and to force businesses to manage data more responsibly. One example of such a regulation is the General Data Protection Regulation (GDPR) of the European Union. In a similar vein, antitrust laws have been put into place to suppress monopolistic behavior and encourage healthy competition, creating a setting that supports consumer choice and innovation.